The Let's Talk Library™

Let's Talk About
Feeling Nervous

Susan Kent

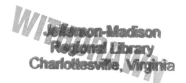

The Rosen Publishing Group's
PowerKids Press™
New York

30 26 4 8 7 7 7

To my dearly beloved Janis and Andrea.

Published in 2000 by The Rosen Publishing Group, Inc.
29 East 21st Street, New York, NY 10010

First Edition

Book design: Erin McKenna

Photo Illustrations by Thaddeus Harden

Kent, Susan, 1942—
        Let's talk about feeling nervous / by Susan Kent.
             p.   cm.—(The let's talk library)
        Includes index.
        Summary: Discusses how new experiences can make a child nervous, how a person physically manifests anxiety, and tips on reducing nervous feelings.
        ISBN 0-8239-5420-X (lib. bdg.)
        1. Anxiety in children—Juvenile literature. [1. Anxiety.] I. Title. II. Title: Let us talk about feeling nervous. III. Series.
        BF723.A5K46 1998
        152.4'6—dc21   98-44976
                                                                              CIP
                                                                              AC

Manufactured in the United States of America

Table of Contents

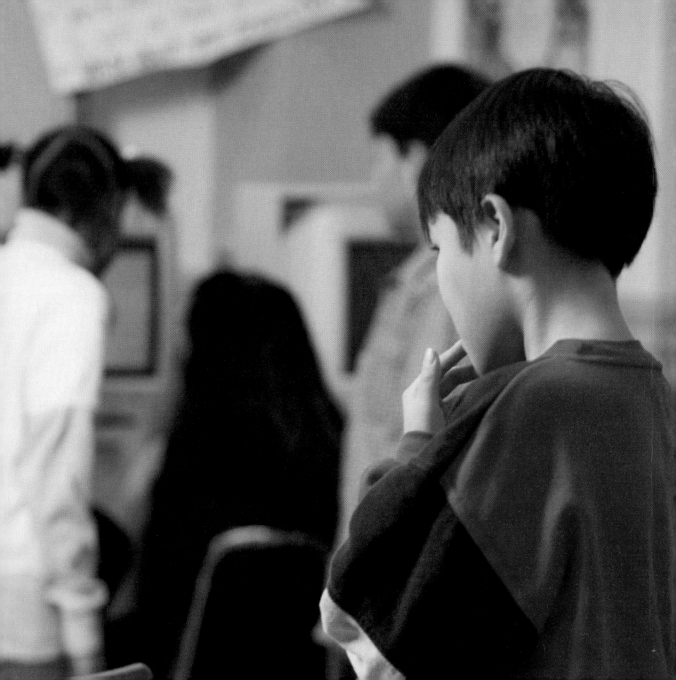

Jesse Goes to a New School

Jesse is nervous. It is his first day at a new school. His family just moved to the neighborhood. He hasn't had time to meet anyone yet. He wonders what the kids will be like. Will anyone talk to him? Will he make new friends? Who will he sit with at lunch? He wonders what the teacher will be like. Will he know the answers if he is called on in class? Being the new boy in school is hard.

It can be hard to meet people on your first day in a new school.

What Makes You Nervous?

New things make most people nervous. Starting new activities and meeting new people can be scary. You might feel nervous when you sign up for a sport you have never played before. Being left with a new baby-sitter may make you uncomfortable. Maybe she doesn't know where to find your favorite books or where you keep your pajamas. Most people feel **anxious** before they take a test. Everyone feels nervous sometimes, no matter how old they are.

Speaking in front of a class makes most people nervous. ▶

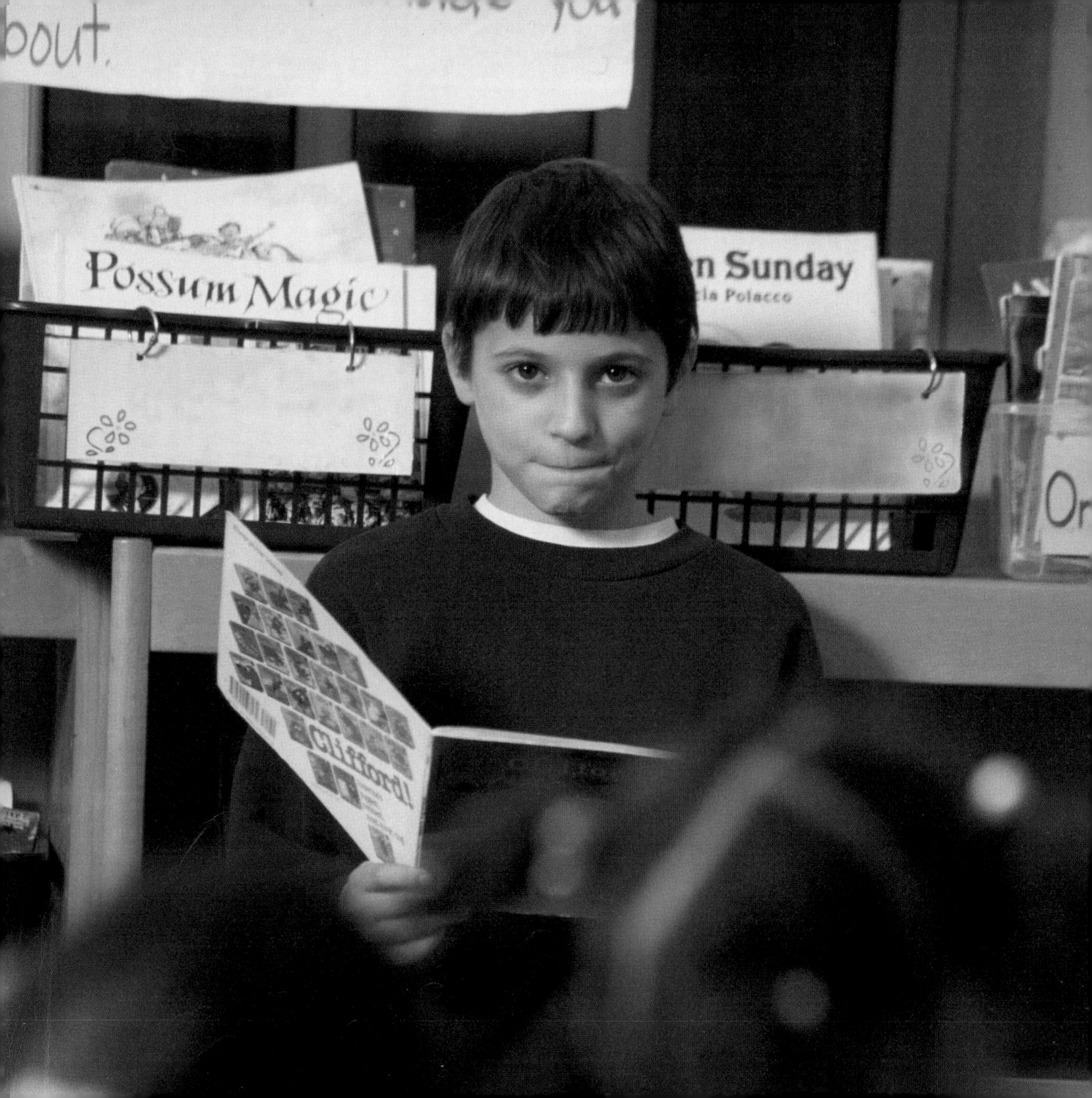
bout.
Possum Magic
Sunday
Clifford!

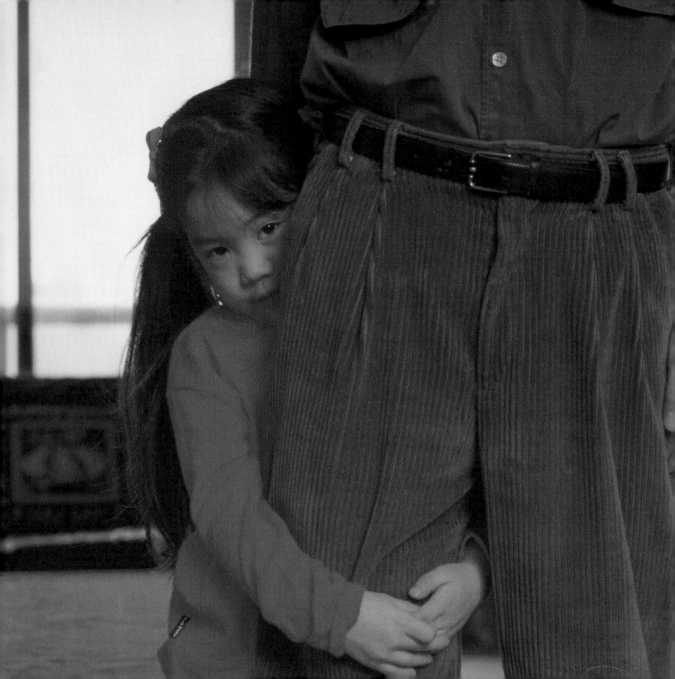

When You Are Nervous

When you are nervous, you might feel like you have a big knot in your stomach. Your heart might beat fast. You may feel shy and not want to talk to anyone. If you try to speak, your words might be so soft that no one can hear you. You may turn red, and your hands may get sweaty or shake. You might get a headache or have trouble sleeping.

These feelings are not fun, but they are very common. They happen to lots of people.

◀ *Sometimes being nervous may make you want to hide.*

What Are Nerves?

Nerves are a special kind of cell found in your brain and all through your body. When something makes you nervous, like going to a circus and hearing a lion roar, these cells pass the message to your body. The message might tell your heart to beat fast, your stomach to ache, or your hands to shake.

When this happens, nothing is wrong with your nerves. They are just telling you that something may be the matter and that you should pay attention to it.

People have nerves in their bodies to let ▶
them know when something is not right.

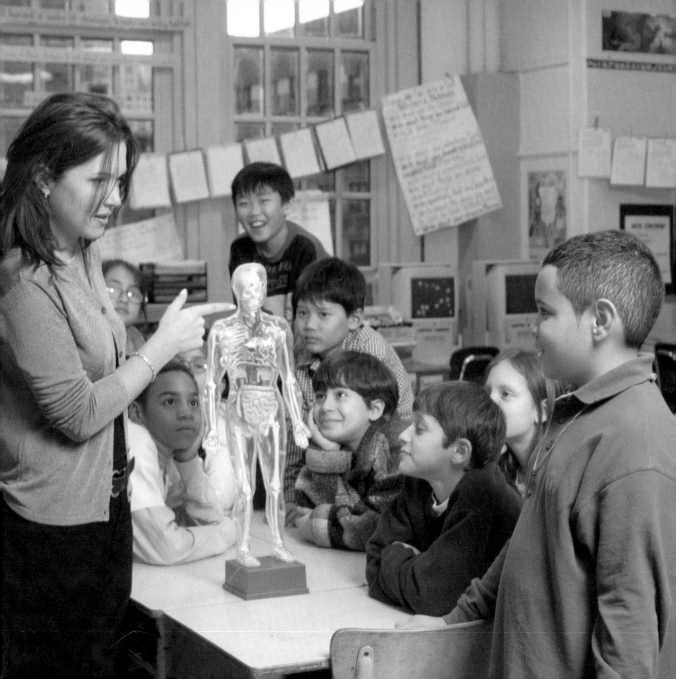

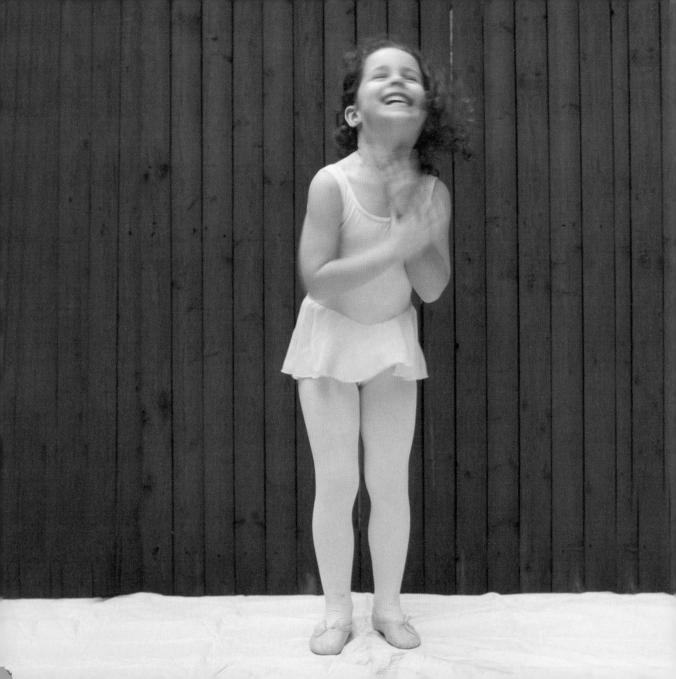

Sophia Stars in a Play

Sophia is happy and excited to be playing the part of Cinderella in her class play. Now the curtain is about to go up. Her parents and grandparents are in the **audience**. Everyone will be watching her. Sophia's heart is beating fast. Her hands are shaking. She is nervous and worried she will forget her lines.

When she steps on stage, Sophia remembers her part perfectly. Her nervous feelings go away once she focuses on doing her best. At the end, everyone claps and cheers.

◀ *Sophia bows and smiles proudly.*

Do Nervous Feelings Go Away?

Nervous feelings can go away by themselves. They disappear when you get used to a new person or place. They go away when you are busy doing something interesting or when you are having fun.

There are things you can do to make nervous feelings go away. One of the best things to do is to **relax**. A quick way to relax is to take deep, slow breaths. Stretch your arms high over your head. Slowly bend down and touch your toes. This is a good way to help yourself feel better.

It's easy to have fun once you are relaxed. ▶

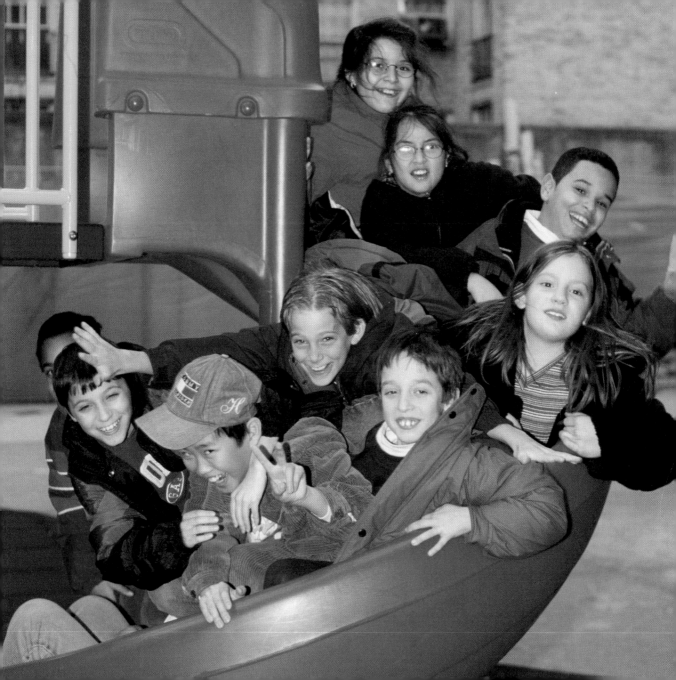

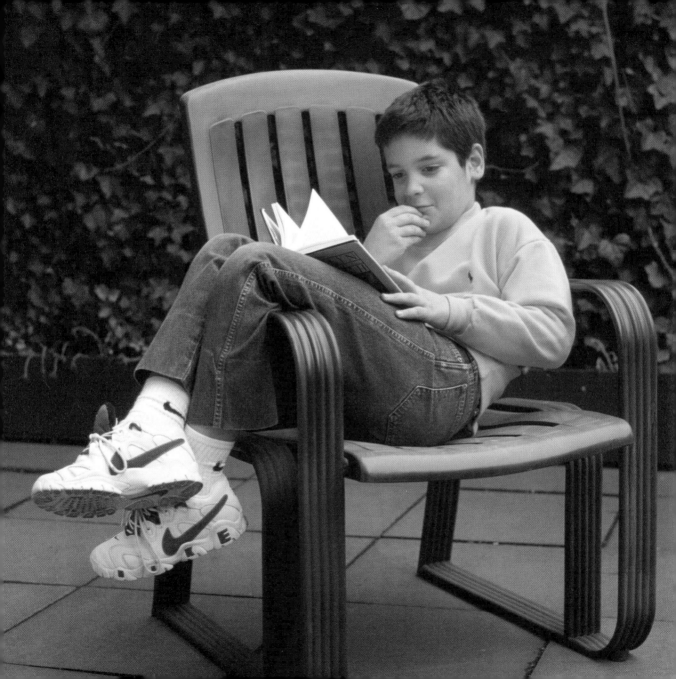

An Exercise to Relax

If you have more time, try this exercise before you do something new or before you go to sleep. Sit somewhere comfortable. **Tense**, or tighten, all the **muscles** in your body. Hold them while you count to six. Then, let them go. Do all your muscles feel loose and relaxed? If not, try to relax any muscles that still feel tight or stiff. When you feel loose all over, imagine you are doing something pleasant and relaxing, like taking a walk, listening to music, or watching the clouds drift by in the sky.

◀ *Some people relax by reading a good book.*

Trying New Things

If you feel comfortable, you won't feel nervous. What can you do to feel comfortable when you try new things? Before you start a new activity, like karate or swimming lessons, visit the place where your lessons will be. Try to meet the instructor. Find out who will be there and what will go on. The more you know about the activity, the better you will feel. Invite a friend to come with you. Doing new things with someone you like can make them easier. You might also want to bring along your favorite stuffed animal or toy.

Having a friend along when you try something new can make you feel more comfortable. ▶

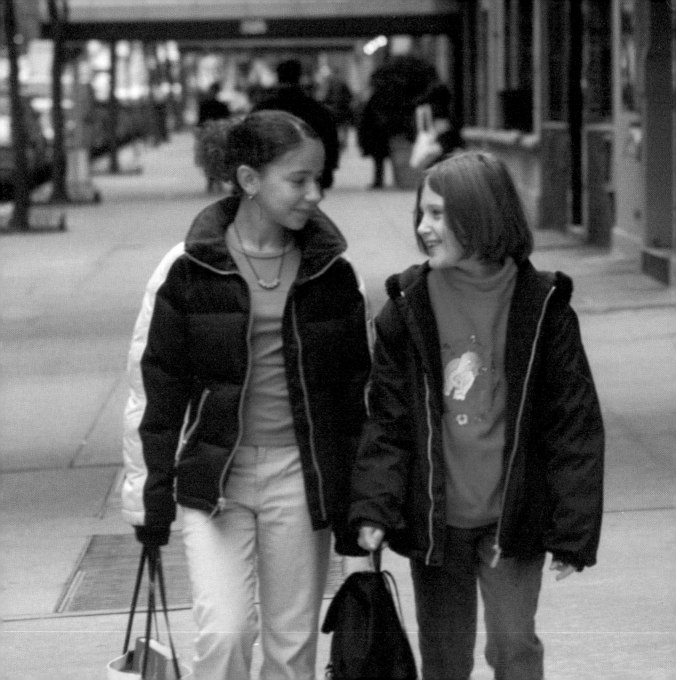

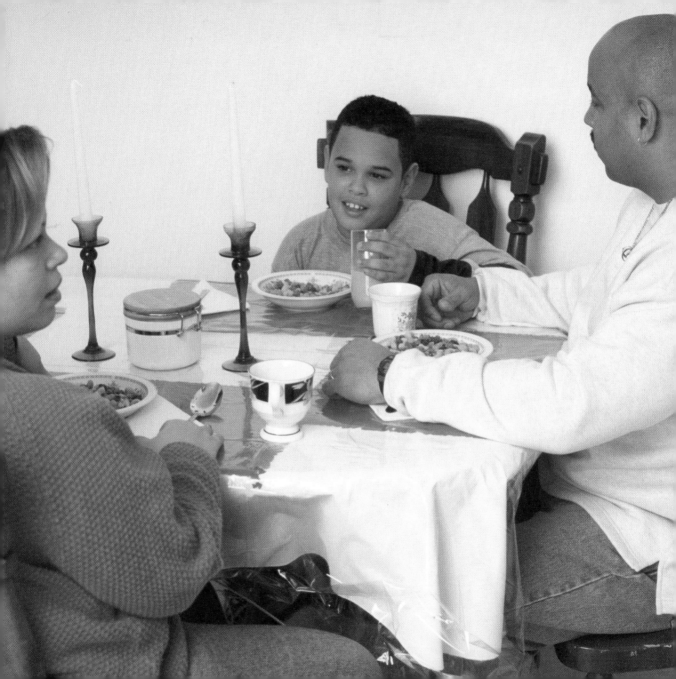

How to Prevent Nervous Feelings

When you are healthy and rested, you are less likely to feel nervous. Be sure to get lots of exercise and plenty of sleep. Eat well. Snack on healthy foods, like fruit and crackers, not candy and chips.

Being prepared can also keep you from being nervous. If you have studied hard for a test, you won't be as worried about how you will do. You will feel more **confident** before a baseball game if you have been to all the team practices.

◀ *Eating a healthy breakfast can help you feel less nervous at school.*

Anika and Howard Go to Camp

Anika and Howard are excited and happy. They are going to camp for the first time. They have already visited the camp with their parents, so they know what it looks like. The camp leader told them what each day will be like and what the rules are. Everything they need is in their backpacks, including their favorite stuffed animals. They also have each other.

Anika and Howard are prepared, so they are not nervous. They are going to have a wonderful summer.

Glossary

anxious (AYNK-shus) Uneasy, nervous, or worried.

audience (AW-dee-ints) A group of people that watches or listens to something.

confident (KON-fih-dent) Believing in yourself and your abilities.

muscles (MUH-sulz) Parts of the body underneath the skin that can be tightened or loosened to make the body move.

nerves (NERVZ) Special kinds of cells found in your brain and throughout your body. Nerves carry messages to and from the brain.

relax (ree-LAKS) To feel loose and to let go of stiffness, tension, or worry.

tense (TENS) To tighten or make stiff.

Index